"Go confidently in the direction of your dreams. Live the life you have imagined."

Henry David Thoreau

"The greater danger for most of us lies not in setting our aim too high and falling short; but in setting our aim too low, and achieving our mark."

Michelangelo

"Keep your dreams alive. Understand to achieve anything requires faith and belief in yourself, vision, hard work, determination, and dedication. Remember all things are possible for those who believe."

Gail Devers

Introduction

Welcome and thanks for picking up this eBook the "Complete Weight Loss Solution". Inside this very eBook I will be revealing to you the exact step by step method I have used to change the lives of many of my personal clients.

If weight loss, more energy and just feeling better and leading the lifestyle you deserve sounds like something you want to achieve, then this eBook is for you.

You'll finally understand why your body does what it does and how you can regain control, your confidence and self-esteem.

You will finally be able to put all the pieces together and make sense of how to lose weight and keep it off long term. And if it does start to creep back on then you'll know exactly what to do to get back on track.

So let's get started.

"The journey of a thousand miles begins with a single step."

— Lao Tzu

Contents

Chapter One Goal Setting

Goal Setting

The most important part of your success is having a clear idea of where you want to go. To get started on the right foot we want to define some goals. But before we do that let's talk about the psychology of goal setting and why it works.

Goal setting is a powerful tool to stay motivated and steer you in the direction you want to go. But often where we dream of being, or what we dream of doing, seems so far away from where we currently are, that the thought of failing to get there is terrifying.

Fear of failure is real and I can guarantee you have felt this fear several times in your life. Not a very motivating state of mind to be in, especially if you are trying to make changes to your weight or your lifestyle.

But if we can separate out our emotions from the goal we are trying to solve then we can look at things in a different way.

For example; do you have a friend who is compulsive eater, or constantly choses the wrong type of partner for a relationship? The problem and the solution are so clear to you. Because you can separate out your emotions and have that outside perspective.

Yet they continue to do the same thing over and over and wonder why they are not getting what they want from life. And often repeat the same patterns over and over again.

The reason you can see so clearly is because you are not affected by any emotions, you are looking at things logically and from that outside perspective. As soon as we add emotions to the way we look at the problem it becomes harder to make sense of it and see the answer that may be starring you in the face.

Also, in terms of weight loss, many people think it needs to be complex. But it is far simpler. Separating out your emotions when setting goals can help get clear on the problems you need to solve.

If your goals aren't clear then you don't know what direction you're going in. This will cause problems for your motivation which is going to fade in and out and not be the burning hot fire that drives you to take action and stick to things when times get tough.

Just define what it is you're after. It might be weight loss, a little bit more energy, fitness, or something else but having something defined, even something small, will be a great start.

Remember goal setting is a process that can and does change over time. Goals are only outcomes of habits. They don't define your success by themselves. So go easy on yourself.

Now the reason why you want to obtain these goals is the next major step to your success. You need to have the reason why clearly defined because that is what's going to really build the solid base for your program.

Many clients I have coached and trained never really made the change to their mindset until 'the why' became so strong and powerful they were able to make the switch. Here's a quick story to explain what I mean.

I once had a story about parent who was a chronic smoker. A pack a day, every day for 30 years type of smoker. They tried quitting a few times over the years but never stuck to it and always ended up smoking again.

Even though they knew it was bad for their health. They were clearly addicted and it looked like it was going to stay that way forever.

Then one day out of the blue the granddad was outside having a cigarette away from the group; it was a family gathering, all the grandkids were there along with the brothers, sisters, aunties and uncle — you get the idea.

When the granddaughter walks up to the granddad and hands him a box.

Inside the box was a packet of those lollies you used to be able get that looked like cigarettes.

Fads I think they were called, but anyway just imagine a cigarette shaped lolly if you've never heard of them before.

And the granddad laughed and asked if they were for him, thinking his granddaughter was playing a trick on him.

But there was no trick, instead a few of the most powerful words he was about to hear that would change his life forever.

The little girl paused, and said softly,

"Granddad, I want you to smoke these cigarettes. They are pink on the inside, so I think they will make you lungs pink again too".

Having heard that the granddad put out his cigarette and from that point on, he never smoked another cigarette again.

He found his why?, His reason for stopping smoking and in that moment a decision was made and everything changed.

I'm sure you'll agree there are 100s of stories like this. However most people don't need this type of event to make a change their habits. For most people they just need the knowledge and confidence to know what to do to get results then they go and do it.

For most people they know they want to change and they have a strong enough why they just lack the knowledge to pull it all together and take consistent action towards the goals they want to achieve.

So the question is? do you have written goals right now? Like I said before. Even if it's just a basic idea of the direction you want to go in that is good enough.

If not it's time to write them down. If you have never written any goals before then here are some tips to get you started.

Think small goals or progress goals. This way if you set your goal of losing 20kgs and you haven't even lost 1kg yet, you may be daunted and scared by the fact that the goal seems so far away.

But could you focus on losing 1kg first? Then 2kgs, then 3kgs and so on.

You see when we break the goal down into smaller more manageable progress goals the big end goal will slowly but surely be achieved. Without all the pressure and anxiety that come with setting goals that seem so large and hard to achieve.

However, this may still happen from time to time but don't worry about it too much as we will be covering how to deal with anxiety and mindset in Chapter 3.

Now that you have written down your goals, let's review some questions. How much do you want to lose? When do you want to lose it by? Let's get a little bit more detailed by identifying exactly what you want to do. Whether it's to be five kilos lighter, or to be a certain dress size again, write it beneath your goals.

This way we are getting super clear on what the end goal looks like. Almost to the point where you can see yourself there already living that goal. You're training your mind to subconsciously move in that direction.

The key is to make sure that it's relevant to you, that it is s going to get you up out of bed in the morning and get you to follow through and take action. Because it's very easy to lose focus of what we want because we build it up in our heads that we want our goal and then we self-sabotage and don't end up achieving the results that we want.

Now that we know what your outcome is and where you want to go let's move onto the next step.

Next Step

We've got our goal, the thing we would like to achieve. Now we need to focus on the how.

How are you going to get what you want? In other words having a plan to achieve the goals you have set. If you fail to plan you plan to fail.

It important to note that the planning part does not need to be any more than 2 or 3 key steps in the very early stages. If you try and change too much and put too much pressure on yourself, you will most likely burn out and become frustrated.

Take it slow and work on one thing at a time.

This is really where having a coach or a trainer to guide you is helpful. Because you are going to have a lot of questions. Even with this guide you will need to keep coming back and reread the chapters that are relevant to you for whatever problem you are facing.

Next Step

A basic way to set goals.

As I mentioned early on, the best way to set goals is to set your outcome goal, i.e. lose 5kgs. Then list all the problems you need to solve to make that happen.

For example, how do I need to eat to lose 5kgs? Ask a question and when you ask questions you come up with answers. It's the way we ask that sometimes sets us up for a negative mindset, but more on that later.

Most trainers, me included, will ask for a deadline for your goal to be achieved. This is a pressure situation. I can guarantee that most of the people I have coached do not like any pressure when it comes to losing weight.

Because most of the time this may be one of the many times they have tried and been unsuccessful at losing any weight. Pressure causes anxiety and stress. Stress can cause your body to be in a state where it wants to hold onto fat, therefore making it very hard to lose weight.

Here's another story to make this point clear.

I once had a client who desperately wanted to lose weight. She was terrified of the gym to the point of severe anxiety; the simple fact of walking into the gym caused her to tense up and the stress she felt was extreme.

Add to this she was desperate to lose weight which further fuelled her stress. So as you could imagine she had set her goals that were very strict right from the start which made her stress levels much higher.

And to top things off work was not very enjoyable at the time so things were tough. As we went on progress was slow and she was disappointed and blamed herself for not being able to lose weight faster.

Things ultimately got to the point where the pressure finally broke her. Her spirit and her motivation died and she completely just let it all go, the training, the diet, work, everything.

It was basically her giving up and resigning herself to the thought that she would never get anywhere. And the thing was she was actually free, all the pressure was gone and she felt like she could breathe again. The weight of the expectations she had put on herself were gone.

And for the next week she just did what she wanted, she took a week off work, ate KFC 1–2 times per day as well as all sorts of other junk food, I guess you could call it a binge. But it was a place where she could find comfort and happiness.

But here is the most surprising thing I have ever heard. All along as I was coaching her, I mentioned over and over about not putting too much pressure on her elf, taking things slowly and so on.

But she had the belief in her head that her losing weight needed to be hard work. Which once you are educated you will know that it isn't true.

She called me on the phone about a week later.

And to my surprise she tells me all that was going on over the last week, the binge eating etc., just the complete letting go of all the pressure.

She was terrified that all the junk food she had eaten over that last week was going to make her weight sky rocket and undo all her hard work in losing the weight that she had.

So she jumps on the scales expecting the worst. And guess what happened.

She had LOST 5kgs!

Let that sink in for a minute, and no I am not making this up. We chatted on the phone and she couldn't believe what she was seeing. But I knew and had seen it time and time again.

The pressure was all but gone from her mindset. She was relaxed and happy. That's why she lost 5 kgs. Even though her diet for that week was terrible it didn't matter because the stress she let go of was the key to her losing that weight.

The point I want to make here is set goals but don't make them so tough that you set yourself up for failure instead use them as a guide to aim for and start to move in that direction that way your weight loss journey become more about lifestyle change rather than achieving something for a time then going back to the old way.

Strategies

Set your goals and write them down.

Break up the larger goals into smaller steps and focus on that step until you've made it.

Remember juggling to many things will end up confusing you and making the whole program hard to stick too.

Identify you biggest trouble area, come up with all the problems and then come up with a few goals based around them. For example, I eat too much chocolate.

Currently I eat five pieces of chocolate a week. My strategy is, "I'm going to cut back my servings to 3 per week" or maybe something along those lines. Make it a strategy that you can implement pretty quick and easy. Or it might be something as simple as, "I'm going to drink more water".

It doesn't have to be rocket science deep down you know what needs fixing so take one thing at a time.

The strategy works better if you try not making too drastic of changes at first. Just identify the three biggest trouble areas and make a conscious effort over the next seven days to make those changes.

Another good idea is to help visualise goals by putting them up somewhere you're going to see them every day. You might do a vision board, possibly on Pinterest. Try making collage or something similar to help keep you focused and get the result that you want.

What you're doing is conditioning your mind to see and change. Visualise what it will be like to already be there. At first you will find this hard but keep reminding yourself of all the good things coming your way and keep up with that positive reinforcement. Your subconscious mind will take on the new beliefs and help to maintain a positive goal setting routine.

A great example is if you ever wanted to buy a car, or a handbag, or a pair of shoes, or something that was a thing that you could buy, but you couldn't afford it.

And you kept thinking about it and thinking about it. Eventually, you visualised the thing you wanted enough that you found a way to get it. Maybe that was by maxing out some credit cards, or not going out with friends, or not having a couple of nights out a week or something else you gave up. This visualisation technique can be used to accomplish your goals.

You need to understand and really be clear on your 'WHY'. Why is it you want to get these results? And keep them in the front of your mind to stay motivated.

Whenever anyone sits down with me for a one-on-one personal PT consultation, that's exactly what we go through step by step. We delve deep into the why.

Now I usually ask the questions and I delve a little bit deeper and yeah, people might say, "Oh, I don't know", for a reason. Then I will delve in, peel back the layers of the onion so to speak, and really get to the root cause of what they want and what's holding them back.

From there we can map out the rest of journey and head in the right direction right from the start. If you don't get that right in the beginning it is really where 90% percent of the people are going to fall down.

Look back on your own life and your own experience with training and losing weight and see if that's not true. Most people stop chasing a weight loss goal because they lose motivation.

You may have been doing it for the wrong reasons, or your reasons were not absolutely crystal clear. Define what you want and why you want it then worry about the planning next. That's the Easy part.

Chapter Two

Diet and Meal Planning

The Complete Weight Loss Solution

If you just want to lose just a little bit of weight or a lot of weight and you are struggling. Diet and meal planning is probably an area you need help with. This section offers some great ideas to help you.

Diet and meal planning are the most important things to consider when dealing with losing weight. You have got to be aware of what you're eating. If you don't know what you're eating, then you really don't realize what you're eating as it could be bad for you and not even know it.

If you are oblivious to the fact of what you're putting into your body, then you can never change it. What I encourage you to do is to download the PDF- Food Diary or join up to my online meal planner to get a start to finish meal plan.

But to get started even just a pen and paper is enough.

For the next 7 days spend time daily filling out your Food Diary religiously. Be sure to include absolutely everything that you've eaten each day for the next seven days.

What you will notice is that by day two or three, your meals will start to get healthier as you go along. Day one may be terrible and day three will be a little bit better.

By the time you get to your seventh day you'll probably find that your meals are exactly where you want them to be. Sounds strange, but it's true.

You will see from reviewing your first few days of your Food Diary just how much rubbish you have been consuming. You will probably wonder why you would be eating this stuff.

You may even probably feel embarrassed to show this diary to anyone. This is when you will notice a change in your diet. And then for the next five days your Food Diary gets increasingly better.

I have had many clients refuse to show me their food diary because they were so embarrassed.

The Food Diary makes you aware of what you actually are eating. You might be thinking why people don't just keep on doing the Food Diary forever. You would think that if you're going to keep a food diary to keep you accountable is going to help you change.

But really what you need to do is learn this lesson now and become aware of your diet. Everybody intrinsically knows what they need to eat and not eat. It has to do with psychology and the mindset that eating is pleasurable and if you're not aware of what you are eating, then you're just going to eat whatever types of food, which may not be the best choice.

 If you have not been doing this for a long time it's hard not to fall back into those old habits and those old routines. It is really important to keep yourself accountable and not just for the seven days, but until you get the results you want.

I can guarantee if you do this for a month straight you'll lose anywhere from three to ten kilos, just by writing down what you're eating. Don't believe me? Then take up the 30 day challenge.

It's free and all it takes is you a pen and paper.

For someone who wants to lose any amount of weight this step works great. Even if you do well for a little while and then you fall off the wagon you just need to get back into the Food Diary again.

Use this information to your benefit and you can always re-correct your course at any time. Keeping your Food Diary is a very important step in this program.

Diet

If you want to lose weight from three to five kilos in the next 21 days, or within the next seven days you could lose one to three kilos if you look at getting rid of things that are intolerant to you.

If you cut out all sugars- processed sugar, all glutens, all dairy, which means breads, cereal, milk, chocolate, all your junk food and drink eight glasses of water daily you would definitely lose weight in that seven day period.

It's basically a simple detox method. Cut the junk and eat the good stuff.

We all know how bad sugar is for us, not to mention how high in calories it is that just puts fat on us almost instantly. Excess sugar converts to fat in the body.

Gluten intolerance is a more of a digestion issue with feeling bloated and messing with your bowel movements. When your body doesn't function properly you get irritated in your large colon and they can become inflamed. Causing bloating and discomfort and poor digestion.

It becomes hard to digest food and you can't get nutrition from your food and you feel tired and run down. Sleep patterns can be disrupted.

Dairy can do the same thing to your digestive system. If you're intolerant to one of these, then you're going to be intolerant to the other because the surface in your small intestine can't absorb nutrients.

They get flattened out and have to regenerate to absorb nutrients and that's all from glutens and dairy. The same can be said of junk foods like chips, candy, sugary foods, anything that's unnatural get rid of them and drink plenty of water.

Continue with your Food Diary over the next seven days. In the free clean eating guide you would have seen a simple list of foods to eat and a sample meal plan. If you have the online meal planner you can just follow that plan.

It can take time for you to realise which foods you're intolerant to or make you feel bloated etc. That's why using a food diary will help you make decisions about the food you've eaten and if there has been any problems like bloating etc.

Just cutting out the foods you suspect of causing a problem. At a later time you can reintroduce them to your diet to see if they're going to affect you. Essentially, you need to do these couple of steps to get started if you're having problems then check out my online meal plan.

Calories

If you're not getting the weight loss you are looking for then you need to look closer at calories. It is important to know about the calorie-in and calorie-out and the basic balance of calories.

You have been told that you don't need to count calories to lose weight.

And yes that is true. But if you consistently can't seem to lose weight then you need to count calories. To get the exact number you need to stick to lose weight.

When you are not losing the weight you want and are following the steps so far, you may need to review your calorie intake and think about some questions.

Like do you need to count calories and will that help you get the results you want. Think of everything in stages and these are the easy introductory stages. When you're getting into calorie counting, that's when you've tried everything else and nothing else is working and you need to get a handle on that.

Calorie counting works and continues to work, and if used in conjunction with everything I'm teaching you here then it REALLY works well.

It's simple; know exactly what you're putting into your body. Then you know how much you need to eat to lose weight.

Meal Planning

Meal Planning is the next step we're going to talk about. Just a couple of simple tips and this always seems to be a bit of a hot topic with people.

Where do you even start? Well there are a few options

Option one. You can search recipes books and the internet high and low to find recipes you like and then also find recipes you actually want to eat. Get out the pen and paper and count all calories, grams of protein and fat. And still not have something that will work for you.

However it is do able. But I like to offer a simple shortcut.

Download the basic to basic clean eating guide if you haven't already and use the sample 7 day plan in that.

Or sign up and join my online meal planner that walks you through the entire process which will save you time energy and of course money. And will get results for you.

It just makes life so much easier.

Other than the actual planning side of things there are other factors to think about.

For some this may be a significant challenge. To make your planning easier consider ideas like bulk buying, having a chest freezer, and most importantly having family support. Be a little bit creative with what you have and can do.

Planning and preparing meals may be easier for singles or couples. Most of this information and guidance can be found in the 'Back to Basics Clean Eating Guide', which is a free giveaway for those that sign up for the email and newsletter.

Get on to the web and search around for recipes you might like, we have a heap of free ones available on the website.

Factors like your budget also need to be considered, family members etc. One big thing I here is that people don't want to have to make two meals and there partners and kids don't support them on their new plan.

Which is a fair concern it won't be easy in the beginning but for example if you can control 80% of your own meals and occasionally eat what the family normally eats and it is outside what your meal plan may recommend?

It's not the end of the world just start out with what you can control and make small steps toward a cleaner meal plan.

Chapter Three

Mindset and Motivation

Mindset and Motivation

These critical steps are an important part of the process. We will spend quite a bit of time on these steps as this is what usually holds people back and can become a roadblock.

Mindset

So far, we've looked at goals, we've looked at diet and now Mindset. Mindset and Motivation go hand in hand. You can't have one without the other and be successful, because your goals affect your motivation.

Your mindset affects your motivation and your motivation affects your mindset. You can be motivated, but without a goal in mind then you have no direction for action. You can have an excellent mindset, and ordinary goals, but without motivation you won't go anywhere.

It is important with particularly weight loss and getting fit and healthy you can't be vague about what it is you want. You must be willing to put the effort out to achieve what you're wanting. You just can't say, "I'm not motivated".

But there is a system to build your motivation.

Motivation

Most people feel like they need TO BE motivated. If you need to be motivated by some sort of outside influence then you may find it hard to stick to a weight loss plan long term.

Your success is determined by an outside factor out of your control.

What we want to teach our selves is to have internal motivation. Motivation that is coming from inside of you not an outside influence.

You can see this type of actions on shows as "The Big Loser" and hear yelling screaming, and carrying on.

Is that motivating, is it motivation? No, it's not motivating at all; it's just holding you accountable for something that you don't want to do to begin with. Ask your self do they look like they are having fun being screamed at.

So, let's flip that around and create motivation that actually drives you closer to your goal. Now if you look at motivation like a table top and you have the legs, if they are not in the proper place they will not hold the table up. You want to look at what will hold your motivation up.

To have motivation you've got to want something like your goal here. Everyone should have goals of things they want to obtain and that's why we took the time upfront to really identify the 'why', the why of what you want.

These are different for everyone and they are critical because all these things layering on top all point to your goal with a bit of Mindset and Motivation.

Mindset and Motivation really form the basis of how you get results. This is the direction you want to move towards. Sometimes you're Mindset and Motivation can be weak, shaky, and not very clear.

Compare this to trying to build a house, how stable and how successful do you think you will be without the proper preparation?

The desire to avoid pain and gain pleasure is the number one principle of motivation.

Pleasure along with fear and pain is generally what motivates people. These types of motivation have to do with essentially values and beliefs. All you've got to do is to recognize that fear and pleasure can move you towards your goal. The question is which one is the one that resonates with you? Is it fear of repercussions or pleasure of something?

Identify which one is the strongest motivator for you. Try thinking back to various examples in your life where you've achieved a goal and how you were motivated.

Where you motivated by the pain of not achieving that goal, or were you motivated by all the feelings of pleasure you would feel by getting the result.

Once you have answered this, you can actually motivate yourself by absolutely taking action and doing it and using what motivates you. Even if, it's only at a basic level that's still good enough.

You must be able to identify this and make it clear in your mind. You don't want to be in the middle with procrastination or into a state of boredom. You need reinforcement to move in your direction of obtaining your goal.

There have been plenty of times where you've been fearful and took action like going to the dentist to get a filling or a tooth pulled out. On the other hand I bet there have been plenty of times when you were seeking pleasure because the outcome was pleasurable with no pain on the way to that goal.

What we really find is that 'fear' is the one that really drives for a lot of people. Particularly, when it comes to losing weight, mainly because they're fearful of dying, having cancer, or being fat, embarrassed, all these things, and eventually what happens is the fear gets so big that you come to the conclusion that you're not going to live this way anymore.

You may be putting off taking action only to have it back fire on you leaving you eventually having to take action.

Generally most people keep repeating the same path without realizing they are in a negative loop by trying to succeed and fail, trying to succeed and fail and get more fearful. Sometimes this loop can cause anxiety and a downward spiral of not feeling great about yourself and what you're trying to achieve. So, how do you break this cycle, how do you stop it?

Recognise The Pattern

One thing you need to do is recognise what's happening. Like a balance of a seesaw, you want to essentially use this fear/pain to get moving, but also you want to make sure they're equal.

We want to balance it slightly towards the side that motivates us the most.

It may be difficult at first to think of examples of pleasure in your life or things you want to move towards, because generally you've been weighted with fear/pain for so long that has hindered any action on your part.

You don't feel as confident and then you generally don't have the energy and the drive or motivation to get to your goal and the cycle repeats it's self. Feel about self. Take no action. Feel even worse about self.

When you're moving towards pleasure your thinking of all the things you will gain by taking that action. Taking a step at a time will help you change your mindset and slowly you can balance out your fear/pain and pleasure to work with you.

Don't let things get out of control and snowball to one side. You want to set it up now so you can easily win. How can you get some quick wins to make you feel good and start to build that decision making muscle.

You're setting your program up so you can have little wins that will build up your positive belief. You will find yourself thinking, I've already done that, what's the next thing? You're building your resilience, your confidence, and your motivation to keep going.

When you start to get towards your goal be sure not to go back, keep moving forward. Take your emotions out of the picture and just think logically. Going back a few steps makes moving forward more difficult. Keep your eye on what is really driving you.

Negative/Positive Balance

Is it more the negative or is it more the positive? Try and keep them equal, because a good balance between the two is going to give you good consistent results.

If you realize that fear is a motivating factor you can use that, but on the flip side you need to be sure to remain positive.

Keep the balance, if you've ever seen people that are chronically upset, down, or just not very happy people chances are they're on the negative side at that time.

Look for those quick wins, build it up slowly, and just start little by little. Remember you're building yourself consciously.

Chapter 4

Weight Loss Psychology

By now you've been going along quite well. Chapter three was going through mindset, motivation and a few other things to think about in terms of getting your results.

You need to realize you have the ability to say no and be assertive and not give into temptation. Don't let other people outside influence your decisions in terms of what you're trying to achieve with your goals and your lifestyle changes.

You need to always keep going back to your goals. As you can see you're building your program step by step. Chances are by now that you've come across some situations where you've had to say no to people or where you felt uncomfortable about asserting your new diet.

What we are going to review is how to say no and not feel guilty about it. Your weight loss goals are important to you in achieving your goals and you're hoping other people around you respect your boundaries and what you're trying to accomplish.

Saying No

Saying no, is if we look at you as a person and you have your sphere of influence, which is where you control your life.

Now, let's introduce the concept of personal boundary. To a lot of people the concept might seem a bit strange of your personal boundaries and personal space. Let's delve a little bit deeper and talk about what actually happens inside your personal boundary and how you should think about it.

This step will help you say no, and not only say no, but hear no as well. Some don't like to say no to people and they also don't like being told no themselves, however, this can be used to your benefit.

Imagine you have a big circle and inside of the circle is your boundary. This boundary is where you have total control over what influences your life. Inside your boundary is 100% in your control. You have the ultimate choice as to what happens within you as a person and this really just basically comes down to what decisions you are able to make.

Everything that's outside of your circle is where you have no control what so ever. This could be the weather, your kids, your partner, how people drive, anything, zero control. However, you can influence certain things to have some control, but ultimately at the end of the day when we're talking about others, you have zero control over what any person does, says, feels, acts, etcetera.

You control you. You can never control the decisions of another person. And factors outside of your control aren't in your control. However you can control how you react to them.

The Personal Boundary

Now, problems occur when you have a weak boundary. When your circle is not complete and has holes or gaps that can cause you weakness in moving forward.

Your boundary is essentially your security and your line of defence against stress and possibly hurt or loss. Stress is based on these two forms – hurt and loss.

It's like the border of a country it and you decide what enters and what goes out. You are your very own customs and border protection for your personal boundary.

Yes, these have happened to us in the past and without control of your boundary, it gets weakened and distracts you from moving forward. What happens when you have a weak personal boundary, the inabilities to say no to people, things, or situations and stress can creep in and out again whenever it likes.

This happens mainly because of the big gaping holes in your boundary. You have no line of defence to help protect your motivation, your mindset, and how you feel about yourself because stress can come in whenever it wants.

You can imagine if you ever been in that situation where people take advantage of you, you're complacent, you let things happen. What happens is that you feel pressured to give in to temptation.

Anytime you have a hole in your personal boundary it is where you want to say no to someone or a situation but you always give in and say yes. Even though you didn't really want to.

To expand a little bit further on your personal boundary is what you control 100%. You actually will have energy or fuel to move forward in the direction of your goal. Your obligation to yourself as a person to be happy is essentially how you can fill your boundary or tank to the brim so you're happy.

This is one way we can think about self-esteem.

You would have to agree that if you were low on energy, low on confidence, low on well-being, low on self-esteem and you could fill up to where you're absolutely overflowing and have more than enough to give away; you have the choice.

But there is a recipe like way to build self-esteem and confidence. And it starts by saying no to those situations that do not serve you.

Essentially, it's the difference between happiness and not being happy and my guess is that everybody likes to be happy.

Let's go back to the holes and the boundary and say you have a container full of happiness, confidence, and well-being, but your container has holes, so your confidence, well-being, self-esteem just falls out through the holes.

Remember, anytime you do feel good about yourself, say you had a good workout, you went to the gym, you followed your diet correctly, or you did all these great stuff then you're filling up your tank.

Patching your holes may be harder with other people's views of, why are you doing that or that's not how you do it.

There could be anything trying to keep those holes in your boundaries open and it's just things outside your boundary that you have zero control over. This constant struggle can leave you depleted with energy, confidence, and self-esteem.

Learning to say no and feel that it is okay is a main step in staying on track. Your psychological resources are worth protecting because this is what makes us happy and feel good. Then you've got the outside influences that can sometimes take you off track.

They may not have any idea of what they are doing, but essentially it's something like- "I brought this cake into work, I know you're on a diet, will you have some anyway?" And you're just like, oh, I don't know, maybe and then you give in.

Generally what happen is if you say no I'm on a diet and I don't want to eat that, you're creating a plug by saying no, and then that person's request is just bouncing off of you. You just keep identifying these situations and keep saying no.

If you've got someone who maybe a little assertive who's not supportive, just stand your ground. Don't let them pull you in; remember you control everything in your boundary. The first couple of times may be hard for you to stay strong and in control; it just takes repetition and practice like building up a muscle.

The more you do this the easier it becomes and you are patching that hole.

You can actually measure how much well-being you are gaining, because when you are saying no to people you're patching these holes and getting your needs met. A good example would be if you have a need to not eat chocolate and yet there is a person in your life that is constantly trying to feed you chocolate.

You say, I have a need to be healthy and happy and I feel like chocolate isn't going to help me do that. You're saying no to that behaviour and you're meeting your need. Try making a list of the needs you've met in your life to feel better, these needs could be anything. And every time you get one of these needs met, you're closing the door or patching that hole on that negative behaviour. You're also building up your confidence, so it's not draining out everywhere like it was before when you had that outside influence coming in and out.

These influences actually don't get in in the first place and you can now fill up on all those good feelings that you get from getting your needs met by saying no. You should be patching those holes on that deal or offer or that outside influence.

We have been using the phrase "outside influence" because it's easier to relate to, but this also could just be your influence too. You might have that battle in your head, where you kind of trick yourself into having something you shouldn't or not going to the gym and then justify it to yourself later. You just need to look at the patterns in your life and realize this is how I'm going to build up my defence by saying no. Essentially, what you're building is a shield.

Remember the power of saying no. It's so simple but it will be best thing you can do for your weight loss and health goals.

Walls in Your Personal Boundary

Now, what you don't want to do is to just block out everything, then your building up a wall. If you ever met anyone who's cold, distant, just has no feelings, no emotion, no friends; chances are they've got massive walls in their personal boundary.

When we have walls up meaning nothing gets in and nothing gets out.

Some people would just put the walls up and not allow anything in or out, which would not help at all in obtaining your goals. Don't go down that path, but just practice by saying no. Think of your boundaries like little doors.

What will happen if you get an offer coming in or a request, well you can choose to open the door and let it in or you can choose to close the door and keep it out so it bounces off you. You will only be able to get to that stage by practicing saying no over and over again, particularly in areas that you know you're weak in.

We want to start thinking in a win/win way. Rather than accepting win/lose deals for example, when you let someone make your decisions or when you fail to say no too people situation or things that do not support your goals.

Recap

Patch these holes and look out for those deals, the psychological deals that make you feel very good about yourself or support you to your goals.

Say no to people, situations or things that don't support your goals.

Just think about how you can patch the holes and how you can operate like a door to let things in and not cut out everything by thinking win/win and rejecting psychological deals that don't serve you.

You need to be able to accept certain psychological trades. Think of it like a border of a country, what country would you be? Are you a country that's free, protects the rights of its people, or are you some third world country that you can just go in and do whatever you want.

This way you can begin to build a new identity based around the new person you want to be.

Understanding how to say no while strengthening your boundary is going to help you stay motivated to protect your mindset and your goals. Allowing you to follow through and get the results that you're after.

Focus on what you can control and let go of the things you can't. Don't waste you precious time, energy and self-esteem to try and change other people or situation.

Practice making more decisions even if they are small at first. Build that decision making muscle and over time it will become easier to identify the situations where you may be tempted or lead of the path towards your goals.

Chapter 5

How to Lose Weight the 9 Step System

The 9 Step System

One of the biggest problems I have found with my personal clients is that they were never taught a system or a frame work on how to actually lose weight.

A step by step method to losing weight and keeping it off that works 100% of the time.

With there being so many different options to lose weight out there it can be hard to decide which is right for you. So that's why I created my own 9 step system to getting any result you want. And it works 100% of the time.

Because as you will discover this system can be applied to you at any time and you be able to see straight away which area you are falling down in.

Pretty much all my clients have told me about their failures on other programs and it always comes back to a missing step in the 9 step system. Not to name any names, but I'm sure after you read this chapter you see what I'm talking about.

How you might be asking? Well it's simple. At any given time we are somewhere along the 9 steps regardless of you are exercising or dieting. Or have never dieted or exercised. It's up to us as individual people to recognize which steps we are doing well and which step we are struggling with because they all affect each other and can be the difference in achieving your goals.

If you think of it like a formula for success then you are well on the way.

Dreams and Goals

+

Mindset

=

Motivation

Diet and Nutrition Plan

*

Correct Exercise Program

+

Testing and Measuring

+

Accountability

X

Action

=

RESULTS

Dreams and Goals   Pretty much the most important thing. If you don't get this right, nothing else below the formula will work effectively.

You should have the right mindset.

Mindset

Motivation

Mindset and Dreams and Goals are also tied together. They back up the three pillars of your Motivation. So without one or the other, you will struggle to stay motivated and get motivated in the first place. Having the right mindset in losing weight is definitely the biggest hurdle that people struggle with. Getting that sorted and giving you the right tips to get that nailed, we'll set you up for the rest of the formula and the success that you are after.

Once we have Dreams and Goals and Mindset and motivation in place, then we can get be motivated and have goals set around a diet plan.

Diet and Nutrition Plan

The Diet and Nutrition Plan is useless if you have poor goals or poor motivation or rubbish mindset. Because it just means you can eat whatever you want and not have the success you are after. You got to have the motivation to eat right to make it truly work

Correct Exercise Program

If you don't exercise, you will never going to lose the weight that you truly want and more to the point, you will never going to keep it off because your body needs to move. It's as simple as that.

Testing and Measuring

What we want to do is we want to have a goal in weight loss, motivated to this weight, have a diet that helps us lose weight, a correct exercise program and Testing and Measuring Process that allows us to make changes to all of the above before they become a problem. Because what most people do is wait until it's too late to try and change something and then there's where they quit.

Accountability Holding yourself accountable and being accountable to all of the above will really keep you on track. Multiply that by...ACTION you are willing to take.

ACTION!

RESULTS This is what you get!!!

Each one of these areas can be broken down further to uncover what is holding you back. And from my experience there is at least 2 or 3 areas that people fall down in or have never even though about until now. Without all of these areas working together this is when we run into the eventual road blocks.

This formula works 100% of the time and it does explain why.

Formula	*If we have;*	*But if we have;*
	Average – not aiming too high, nothing excites you, you will have...	
Dreams and Goals		*Incredible*
+		
Mindset	Average	*Incredible*
=		

	Average	
Motivation		*Incredible*

Diet and Nutrition	Average	
Plan		*Incredible*

*

Correct Exercise	Average	
Program		*Incredible*

+

Testing and	Average	
Measuring		*Incredible*

+

	Average	
Accountability		*Incredible*

X

	Average	
Action		*Incredible*

=

	Average	
RESULTS		*Incredible*

It's as simple as that! Question is, ***are you doing everything AVERAGE or doing everything incredibly?*** Chances are if you reading this report, you are probably leaning towards the average or the poor side in a number of those areas.

Another way of explaining this idea is the formula below

BE	Who are you willing to be, as a person
X	
	The person you are and the action you are willing to
DO	take.
=	
	This is the formula, breaking it down to as simple as
HAVE	that.

If you;

Be Average, Do Average, Have Average Results

But if you;

Be Incredible, Do Incredible, Have Incredible

The System Works, Whether You Use It or Not

Everybody is doing those steps at every point in their life. The question is, are you doing it on a high level or at a lower level? And if you are overweight, Chances are you have fallen out in many of those areas.

So What Can You Do About IT?

Many People Fall Down In one or many of These Areas.

You have to start at the Top and work Your Way Down. –You can't fix it from the bottom up. It's a top down proposition and I'll explain why.

It's the only path to Succeed! – And long term success at that.

Step 1 – Dreams and Goals	If you don't have these clear, you are doomed from the start. Why? Because, they are the Corner Stone of Motivation. Motivation is the biggest buzz word you will hear in fitness and training. It's the most important because you have to get out of bed in the morning and you got to want to do it, you got to have enough reasons why to get started. The problem of people is how to get started in the 1st place. The more motivated you can make yourself, the easier the next 6 steps are going to be. The right mindset can only be achieved when you have clear goals. If you can't have the two working in unison (Goals and Mindset), you will not get the results you want. You cannot hit what you cannot see.
Step 2 – Mindset	The correct mindset will always move you forward.
Step 3 – Motivation	Dreams and Goals X Mindset = Motivation They work together to form unstoppable confidence. People with uninspiring goals, and a rubbish mindset =

95% of people unmotivated.

Account for a huge part of your success. Some say up to 90%, others say it's a huge part. You can't have one without the other. **There's no way around it.**
You cannot cheat.

If you cannot accept this, then you will never get anywhere.

If you are going up against your own mindset in saying that I can lose weight without eating correctly, then in the long term, you will fail as simple as that. You have to accept the fact that you have to eat well and you need to do it consistently to have any sort of a long term success. If you are not willing to accept this, then there's nothing we can do for you. You have to accept it and you have to know it. This is the biggest hurdle in diet that people face because they think they can get away in eating junk food and justify it by doing extra exercise. You can outeat your exercise with a bad diet.

Step 4 – Diet and Nutrition   Just be careful.

Equally as important with diet. The Confusion around exercise is mind blowing! Being a personal trainer, you come across all sorts of stories people think to fact but the sad thing is it couldn't be further from the truth and usually the simplest thing is usually the right thing. People have been bombarded with marketing messages, infomercials, and friends and family, everybody is an expert on exercise. Learn from a professional to cut through all the rubbish and get yourself started on the right track.

People are out of touch on what works and what doesn't. That's the biggest problem I face in exercise. People don't want to do the exercise that will contribute to their result and they want to fight that process.

Step 5 – Correct Exercise Program

People get into the trap of doing the same thing, day in and day out. If anybody knows anything about exercise, that's the worst thing you can do to your body. Especially when you want to achieve fat loss. One of the most neglected steps. **Know your starting point.** You got to know your starting point. How could you ever know you have changed something? If you have gotten better or worse.

Step 6 – Testing and Measuring

You cannot change what you do not measure. If you are trying to lose weight and you don't know what you are eating exactly, or you don't know how much weight you have lost or gained, or where you started from, your motivation and confidence will go down the toilet because you really just don't know where you are going.

You'll never know what's working or not working.

You need feedback to change your approach. This is where your personal coach comes in, personal trainer, to give you feedback and point you to the right direction. When you are doing your own thing, you cannot see the forest from the trees. It's very hard to get an outside perspective when you are always on the inside.

Keep you on track. Don't accept excuses. Everyone should have a little urge time.
Push you to do a little more each time.

A mentor, a coach, an Expert. This is what you need.

Step 7 – Accountability   Probably the greatest thing you'll do for yourself if you try to lose weight.

How much are you willing to do? How much are you willing to take on? How bad do you want it? **The**

Step 8 – Action **hardest step, killing procrastination. Procrastination-**

It's the opposite of taking action. It's safer and comfortable to do nothing than to take action. What we want to do is flip it over its head.

Use baby steps.

Build your action taking muscle!

Start yourself small and work your way up bigger and bigger and bigger, until you are so consistent that you feel wrong if you don't take enough action. You actually feel bad doing nothing. To move you more into action more often to help you maintain your results.

This is the result of the other 8 steps. You can see how they all affect each other.

If you've failed in the past, now you cans see where. If haven't had a good diet, no amount of training, no amount of mindset, no amount of accountability is going to fix it, If your diet is rubbish. If you had a great diet, but you didn't exercise, you can see why, you if didn't maintain your results and vice versa, if you have fallen down on those areas on the things you need to work on, most of all, remember to start from the top down.

Step 9 –
Results

After looking through this 9 step system you might find that you can relate to some of the areas if not all of them. This is the steps I take my personal clients through to uncover all their hidden road blocks. But just being aware of the system and the steps will help you realise your challenges might be.

Just remember the system works, and if you constantly find yourself hitting the same roadblocks now is the time to address them and come up with a plan to overcome them.

The weight loss mindset is a really important part of your loss journey. So much of why we fail or have problems when it comes to losing weight can be traced back to our mind sets. But really what does mind set even mean and how can you use it to get what you want?

So why is it and how is it that these underlying beliefs about ourselves sometimes control how and dictate why we take action and why we fail to follow through. On the things we really want to achieve and know will make a positive difference in our lives, often without us even realising what is happening our minds and body's just seem to cruise on autopilot

In my opinion mindset is really in a nut shell what we think about, and how we think about it. The "It" being whatever is causing a problem, or a desired goal which we are aiming for yet things are happening around you and cause you to get taken of course, or cause stress or even cause you to give up and stop trying.

But on the flip side mindset can also be positive leading you to break through challenges and get success, whether that be going to the gym 3 times per week or not giving into a temptation like eating chocolate or some other junk food.

It's sad to say that negative mind set is the far more common mindset we run into, and I can tell you everybody at some stage will have a negative mindset; it's just a fact of life. But when we apply this to body image, health, fitness and feeling good you ask people about such things and you can bet you will get some pretty strong beliefs about it. Some people will love and some people will hate it. This is their mindset to leading and living a healthy life.

The question is what is yours? And it's easy to find out. On any given day you talk to yourself (in your head of course, no you're not crazy lol) and you ask your self-questions or you fixate on a problem and for most people if there is a problem or they are struggling with something most people don't like at this and say to themselves "Yippee! Another problem I have to deal with today, this losing weight thing is so much fun! I love working hard and not seeing any results! This is great!"

I have a never seen this or heard this from anyone, if they did then they would be crazy!

At the first sign of a challenge it automatically triggers a belief about what it means to you usually a negative one

Example

"I just can't lose weight" = I'm a failure

"This is too hard" = I'm a failure

"I keep trying but nothing ever seems to work" = I'm a failure

They idea of being a failure (negative belief) is the one that quite often

Drives you back down to where you subconsciously believe you deserve to be

Think about that for a minute, no matter what I say or anyone says about you – even if it is positive, there is a deep seated belief in you about what you deserve, how happy you feel about yourself, how confident and also what your are capable of. No matter what. This is you, your absolute core belief about yourself.

Now if your core belief about your self is that you are a failure, think about where did this come from? And what is it holding you back from and how is it effecting you?

Because this is why all the fluffy pump you up motivation in the world won't make a difference, because deep down you still believe that where you are, what you have and you believe about yourself is truly what you feel like you deserve.

So how do you change it? Good question. As you can imagine its not easy – if it were there would be millions of successfully happy people out there that wanted to change, decided to change and then they did it. But we all know it doesn't work like that it's more like the picture below

Success on any level is never a start line path to your goal, but the key to getting there is controlling your mindset and making your focus on the positive. So here are some simple steps to get started

1. Keep track of your thoughts each day and notice where your focus is positive or negative, this alone will help you notice any patterns in thinking

2. If a same feeling or belief pops up sit back and look at why you're feeling this way, is it a person, a situation something outside of you that is causing these feelings to pop up

3. If you can look find a source of a negative belief about yourself look at make changes, if it's a person try and let them know, if it's a situation make sure you remove yourself or distance yourself to give yourself time to adjust

4. Find someone to talk to about it even if it's just a friend let them help you explore how you feel because awareness is the key to helping build a strong mindset

5. Don't rush it just little by little each day start to build up a new belief about yourself and frame it in the positive light, and over time gather new evidence that makes it stronger

Chapter 6

Lifestyle Factors

Lifestyle Factors

How to use lifestyle factors to your advantage and the other factors that can prevent you from getting your weight loss results.

Some major lifestyle factors are the things like work, family, or just your environment. There are probably a few other things that can be viewed as lifestyle factors that might be considered major factors. Like, how do you spend your time and who do you spend your time with? Now, if we look at a little pie chart being equal, but it's not quite working out that way.

With 24 hours in a day, how much of your day is balanced? You probably have areas for your pie of work, play, and rest. In a perfect world you would have an equal third of pie for each of the three areas.

Our job taking up a third of our day, you play through a third of the day, and you rest for a third of the day. In reality though with society, our work takes up most of our time, which leaves just a little bit for rest. What's the problem with that? Well, you're out of balance.

This is essentially what lifestyle factors are and balancing these factors that's comfortable for you. How can you make the best changes and implement strategies that are actually going to help you keep balance in your life.

We all have busy lives, you've got a list of things to do, run to school, get groceries, house work, your job, gardening, and other obligations. Now, add exercise to your list. Where is that on your list? Is it number one, or is it number 100?

Priorities

For some exercise and eating well is already a priority in their lives. On the other hand for other people, exercise, diet, lifestyle, and fitness are not priorities on their list. A lot of people go to work and can't wait to get to the gym in the afternoon, whereas as others are the opposite.

Now, where do you see you fit into this scheme of things? You've got to get exercise and learn about the lifestyle that should be high on your list of priorities. This is the next step if you're going to have long term success and actually want to change your life.

Of course, if it doesn't come naturally for you, that's okay at this point. That's something you can change over time and exercise in the 9 step system is ranked lower on the list. Because it doesn't help if everything above it isn't working.

You want to change that belief to maybe more exercising or something higher on your hierarchy of needs. The way you're going to do that is to start with a new belief. Changing your belief means changing your behaviour.

You will see that your old and new beliefs will be in conflict with each other. Generally, what happens is people go back and forth between the two. You want to exercise more or make a lifestyle change. It all boils down to belief and the "I am" statement. I am.... I'm too busy, I'm too tired, I can't do it, I'll do it tomorrow, I'm okay, etcetera.

And that's fine for you to be like that. However, the only thing is when you're in conflict between these two beliefs, it's like you want to have your cake and eat it too. You want both, but you can't have both, because the bigger one of the two is always going to win out in your decision making.

Some people find making lifestyle changes easier when training and/or working a partner, family or friend. Going through these steps with someone that will assist in keeping you accountable and give you someone to talk to and share this journey with will make your changes easier.

If we look at a perfect day it would be 1/3 work, 1/3 rest and 1/3 play.

If you look at the lifestyle pie again, where would you rather be? A lot of people don't want to spend all their time at work or is that just another excuse? Do you think maybe that you might use excuses to stop taking action and be out of balance? If you're living your life in the way that work, rest, and play are pretty equal, then you're pretty balanced and happier with more energy.

Work can be so demanding and mentally draining that it's very hard to follow through with exercise and workouts.

Thinking about exercise that fits in with your lifestyle is all you need to worry about. Workouts don't have to be all indoors, but it is important to find exercises that fit in with your lifestyle that isn't going to add stress to your life.

In Chapter 7 we will be reviewing stress and how to avoid it. Stress is pretty important and has a huge impact on everything that we've covered so far. Not just exercising, but trying to find the time to fit it in can be stressful too. Various factors can get in the way, like friends and family. Your friends, family, and co-workers are the people you spend most of your time with.

So, essentially you're a reflection of these people that you spend your time with. So if your friends, family or co-workers are overweight people, unhealthy and uninterested in health and fitness, you will find that this may hinder any lifestyle changes you want to make. Being around more people that are looking at the same goals will help you in getting motivated and staying on track.

Reflect back on Chapter 4 of your personal boundaries. On the flipside when you get around people that are supportive and positive about health and fitness and you too are positive about health and fitness and then add three other people.

Whether it be people you make friends with at the gym or people you go and exercise with or whoever might be. You may not even realize this is going on. What you have done unconsciously is created this little group together whereas the energy is shared between all.

Then you can actually take this group energy and bring it into your boundary and fill yourself up with confidence.

If you have ever had a time in your life where you've been upset or felt down about something and you go and chat with a friend and then you feel better. Same thing applies to your fitness and getting around people that are positive, it rubs off on you.

This concept does not just apply for fitness, if you want to make changes you need to get around people that are like-minded and already taking action. It's very hard for you to succeed if you've got people pulling you back or dragging you down.

Rather than cutting them out of your life or cutting them back, just realizing that it has a huge impact on your results and your ability to do what you need to do is a major realization.

So, an assignment for this chapter is to look at your lifestyle. List the top five things that are holding you back and these might be very similar to your goals that you set in chapter 1.

And now that you're halfway through working through your goals and taking some action you can really start to identify what may still be holding you back and finding out what these limiting lifestyle factors are.

As in chapter 1 you want to identify them, list them out, and then come up with some strategies on how you can change them. Next, look at how you're spending your time; are you happy with how you're spending your time?

Are you making time for exercise? Is it number one, or is it number 100? Where does it sit for you? If you need to make a change, go through the exercise, identify it, try it with the least amount of stress and incorporate it into your routine.

Time Management

This all comes back to time management. How do you plan your day, have you got everything set out? Like when you're making your meals, when you go to the gym, when you go to work, etcetera, etcetera.

Have you got it in your calendar? Treat it like an appointment and then just follow through, especially if you've got a busy life.

Treat all you weight loss related tasks as appointments with yourself. So you can always give them the time and attention they need.

That's really all you can do. If you're not getting the results or making the time, go back and look at your beliefs again and ask yourself the question, is there something I need to work on in that area and then just make it a focus.

Move forward with everything up to this point. All things being equal, if your lifestyle gets in the way, you're never going to have the time to take action on all the stuff that you've learned so far. But if you do make time, then it's going to reward you and you'll be fine.

Chapter Seven Yo-Yo Diets

This Chapter I will reveal to you what actually happens to your body in yoyo dieting, the warning signs, how to avoid it, and really how you can protect yourself from the rebound weight gain associated with yoyo diets.

Yoyo Diets

What are Yoyo Diets and how can you protect yourself by recognizing the yoyo diet's cycle? You need to really understand what's going on with your body when you get on a crash diet or a quick fix diet that doesn't yield long term results.

What actually happens in terms of calories and how your body reacts to calorie deficits? If you've ever been on a diet where you have a rebound of weight gain or a feeling that you just can't stick to a diet, we will illustrate what is actually going on.

Let's look at the calories in versus the calories out. Calories may not be that important in having a healthy diet, but what's going on at the various stages is. This particularly example will give you a good base to look at until you learn enough to know what you should be eating and how much. You will understand more about the sensation you get when you're full and when you've had enough while balancing at your energy levels.

Calorie Example

Let's use a 1600 calorie example and a female as an example due to the fact that most females have fewer calories than males to maintain their body weight. We have 1600 calories here and say she weighs 80 kg. She won't gain or lose theoretically at that 1600 calories mark. Let's call her Jill. So Jill decides she is going on a diet and lose weight.

She picks up new ideas from one of those magazines and some celebrity diet that encourages a crash diet disguised as a quick fix. Now she is happy that she has a celebrity diet that worked for that celebrity. She's going to start the diet and she decides to go on a drastic change of eating.

So, she's been eating normally throughout her diet and everything stays the same. With seven days in this new diet, she's turned her whole level upside down, eating whatever is called for in the diet that encourages really fast weight loss.

What will happen is usually the calories of that diet are going to drop drastically. Over this time period, she's dropped and she may have lost three to five kg straight off the bat and then, what she's done is reset.

She's reset her maintenance calorie level. So all Jill is thinking is yeah, seven days later, three to five kilos lighter, she is absolutely stoked. However, what she's done is just reset her maintenance level from the 1400 to the 1200 calorie mark. She keeps going on with the diet for another fourteen days.

Feeling pretty happy with herself as she's getting some results. Next, what happens is she starts to get a little bit less of a drop, maybe just another one to two kg. Now, she's down to the 1200 region and her new maintenance is now1200. So she has gone from 1600 maintenance with no weight gain or no weight loss.

She has dropped down to1400 in seven days and she's lost that three to five kg straightaway in that seven day period. She's gone along for another seven days with a little bit less weight loss and more around the 1200 mark losing one to two kilos.

She's thinking okay, that's just the initial weight loss. This is starting to get a little bit harder now, let's say her goal is to lose fifteen kilos, which isn't unreasonable by any means. But now she's two weeks in and she's down to six kilos, that's pretty standard for a fresh diet that promises fast results.

Jill thinks this is perfect and awesome! By dropping her food a little bit more because she didn't get as much weight loss this week but she is almost halfway to her goal. So Jill thinks that eating less now, and before we move on obviously, we need to keep in mind that she's down to the 1200 calorie maintenance.

So far her thought process seems right. Let's get to the 21 day mark of three weeks in. By now what she does is drops down again and only loses 500 grams to one kg. She is three weeks into this diet and this was a really hard slope because she was really starting to get lower in calories and now she is down to a new maintenance level of 1000 to 800 calories.

Her idea is now that she has lost that initial weight loss, she thinks if she eats less again then she'll lose more. This is what most people assume that if they eat less they will lose more weight.

The nine to fourteen day mark is starting to get tough and she pushes herself and is starting to really struggle in the gym three to five times a week eating close to a thousand to 800 calories. She is starting to get really, really tired, struggling to maintain the weight loss and she's thinking "I'm dieting harder, not eating as much, doing more and more and more, trying to do it in a faster time frame.

She doesn't realize that she is getting dangerously close into starvation territory. This is really where you don't want to be. This low calorie count can cause a lot of health problems this is the danger zone. You can't stay in the danger for very long, you may experience irritable, anxiety, be upset all the time, and you just don't feel very good.

Starvation Response

Jill has already dipped in into the danger zone area going from 1600 calories all the way down to 1000 to 800 within a matter of just three weeks. Because she's lost three to five plus another two plus 500 grams, so that's seven to eight kilos combined she's still feeling pretty good like this diet's working.

She feels that she has lost so much weight, but now she is really struggling and finding it hard to keep on track. She still decides to go another week. Generally, most people won't last three weeks on these types of diets. Now she is at day 26, so another five days in. She's gone from the top to a really low calorie range.

Down to 800 calories and didn't lose anything, zero, big fat zero. Now she's going to try and maintain that. If she was really committed, this is what a lot of body builders would do to get really lean and lose a lot of fat.

This takes a lot of mental power to stay down and it's not very healthy to stay down for a long period. These fad, crash, yoyo diets to new people can be dangerous not knowing and realizing what's going on with each one of these steps. They just keep going by eating less and less, while working harder and harder and getting less result.

So Jill is failing with this diet, a big fat zero. She tries it for another three days, but this time she's ravenously hungry, stressed out, can barely even make it through the day because she's so hungry. When she finally gets to 26 days, if she makes it that far taking this crash course she realizes this is a crap diet and she's going to go back to the where she was.

The Rebound Weight Gain

Let's bounce back to the 1600 calories no weight loss, no weight gains. She went from 800 to 1000 calories and shot right back up to almost two times to what she was over that three week period and the body thinks it is surviving at 800.

She thinks she's not going to gain any weight. All of a sudden she's got two times as many calories in her body that need to be used and the body is already in stress. When you're in stress, you store fat and your body looks at those extra calories.

Now the body puts that into fat storage for the next time when it's in the starvation situation, a natural survival mechanism. When you have a low calories intake the body thinks it's dying and stores everything it has. Then all of a sudden you will shoot back up to two times the calories you've been used to over that three week period.

Usually it's a lot more than that because there's a compensation effect where the body will overcompensate and make sure that it is full and has plenty in reserves for next time you go through the yoyo diet.

No one intentionally sets out to destroy their body when trying to lose weight. Generally though, when you follow a fat diet or a crash diet that's the process it takes you through and you don't really realize what's going on and then all of a sudden, bang and that's why you get poor Jill.

So she's lost that 7 kilos and then she's come back up so within a week or two, she's put on that weight again plus probably an extra three to five kg's, maybe more depending on how severe the yoyo effect was.

Maybe she just really got depressed and down and started emotional eating which made this even worse. Jill sort of comes down, gets back into a routine and then starts to bring herself back down to a normal rate, but chances are she's probably reset her metabolic rate, which set her at 83 to 85, possibly more kilos.

So this whole endeavour has left her with an extra five kilos for all this pain and suffering and this is how a yoyo diet works.

Going through these stages you can see how hard it is when you get down and how hard it is to stick it out and then to have the weight go back up. That's where it hits you the worst and then you carry that around.

Jill goes away for a few months feeling sorry for herself, a bit disheartened because she got sucked into this yoyo diet from the magazine. Maybe down the road she goes, okay, I'm ready for another crack at it.

She's ready to go again because she's not happy with her body and so she finds the next diet to jump into and repeat the same process. All over again without realizing what's going on and that's what yoyo diets do, up and down, up and down, over a period of years and each time you add a little bit more weight, add a little bit more, add a little bit more. You get the idea.

You might start out leaving high school at 80 kilos and over a period of ten years, you could be a hundred plus kg's, no problem at all. It's easy to put on weight over ten years, but it's hard to lose when you're constantly in this yoyo diet predicament.

Chapter Eight Stress

Why Stress Matters

This chapter we're going to talk about stress and why it's important to understand and realize that stress can put on the brakes on everything that you've being doing well on up to this point. If you are stressed, you can be eating right, sleeping right, training right, doing all the right things, but if your stress isn't under control then you going to have problems with your results. When we look at stress as a whole, we can divide it into six different categories.

Physical Stress

We've got Physical Stress, which is the stress we put on our actual physical body. Meaning stress through exercise or not enough exercise, working too much, being sick or we might even be injured. Physical stress that is put onto your body can be good and bad, we do need both. So exercise can be good and exercise can also be bad.

Be sure you've got the right ratio depending on how much energy you have and how much you can take. This is initially where we start. Exercises in Week 5 is where we started really getting into them, because we needed that four weeks of preparing and recovery to get everything set up and on the right track.

Chemical Stress

The chemicals in our food, what we put onto our skin and pollution are another type of stress. These things all add to the spectrum and generally if you have a diet that is pretty free of pesticides, then there is not a major worry here. If you use things like deodorants and some perfumes and products that contain toxins and heavy metals that soak into your body, then there is cause for chemical stress.

Electromagnetic Stress

Electromagnetic Stress happens when being around TVs or other things that can cause electromagnetic pollution. There is good Electrometric Stress which can also become a problem. The good stress in that regard is like moonlight and sunlight. Due to their magnetic field on the earth, which helps things grow and live. Plants, animals, grass, trees, and sounds are essential, but in our modern world because we're so busy with our computers and our phones and so on can be too much.

Mental Stress

We have Mental Stress, which is the big one. Your mental outlook and mental health have a very big link between them. Here is a quick story about a previous client. She's trying to lose weight, but didn't get any results.

Her failure was because she didn't do all these other steps correctly and was very reluctant to really get a hold of the process. Then she flipped out, had a bit of a melt down and just said, "I'm not doing any training".

She went away from the program for a little while. After about a week off work and just totally resigning herself through that stress and that feeling, she ate KFC and junk food. Then she started feeling sorry for herself and she jumped on the scales. Keep in mind that she had just totally let go of all the pressure of trying to lose weight and changing her life, so it was just like a lot of weight that had been lifted off of her shoulders.

To reward herself she just fell back into old habits, but the key point is that the stress was removed from her life. She ate all these junk foods, jumped on the scales and she was actually five kilos lighter than when she was a week ago.

She rings me up on the phone and tells me "you'll never believe what happened" and just couldn't believe she was five kilos lighter. I could tell in her voice and her body that the stress that she was feeling was gone.

Nothing else had changed, she was eating crappy food and not looking after her body, but because that stress was gone her body it was just like thank you now I can relax. This is hugely important and very powerful to understand and recognize that if you are stressed, you're not going to go anywhere in terms of weight loss. This is physiologically impossible.

Nutritional Stress

Nutritional Stress can happen of course by an unhealthy diet. Eating good food versus bad food is pretty much self-explanatory.

Thermal Stress

Thermal Stress is just basically hot-cold, making sure you look after that respite. What your body does is it summates and adds all these stresses up into one big stressor. Your body doesn't recognize that you are physically stressed today or that you're going to be chemical stressed. It doesn't work like that; your body summates into one big stress picture and then at the bottom is where stress weighs in.

Generally, what happens is if you weighed too much on the bad side or the good side, ideally, you want to be in balance. You want to have a good amount of bad because that singles off the good and then you have good balance. You don't want to have the good all the time, but you need these things to keep you alert and active.

It's all about balance. Most people are balanced onto the bad side with signs of fatigue, depression, anxiety, low energy levels, just feeling tired all the time, not a lot of growth, not a lot of repair. Not a lot of happiness, which is on your parasympathetic branch of your nervous system. So, that's something to keep in mind with that.

What we're going to do for Week 8 is download the exercise. Review the stresses and write out some of your top stresses and how they might be affecting you. Start by writing down your top three to five stresses and we will review some strategies on how you can overcome them.

Strategies

You've identified your problem and stresses, now we are going to make a plan or a strategy to help to remove or minimize the stresses that you're feeling. We come back to Week 4, about saying no and your mindset around this. Your barrier is your barrier to your stress as well. Let's review particular strategies or instances where you have stressful situations and then how to obviously avoid them, so you're not adding extra stress on your body.

You want to make a plan, for instance you're stressed about work. What about work, are you stressed about? Is it deadlines? Is it you haven't got enough time, you're doing too much work? You just need to sit down and reflect on what this might be. You might need more hours to do a job or you might need to get someone in to help you or you might need to offload tasks.

You might need to have uncomfortable conversations with your boss. Are you prepared to take the burden off the stress of the situation onto yourself or is there a way that you can sort of brush it off or give it to someone else and not have to worry about it? Obviously, you've got responsibilities that you need to worry about, so it's not going to be practical to get rid of everything. But there's going to be some areas where you can tidy up and make some changes in that area particularly at work. Work stress can be such a huge problem for a lot of people.

Let's look at play and relaxation. Do something that makes you happy at least once a week, maybe even twice a week. Do it more if you can, whether it's catching up with a friend or watching a movie or chilling out, whatever it is, make sure you set aside time to do that activity. Some might enjoy doing some craft, maybe in the garden, playing a video game or anything. Whatever it is for you, try and take the time out, acknowledge that you are doing these for relaxing reasons and then this is going to help balance you with your stressful situations.

Nutrition is obviously a huge part of this. Yes, you are what you eat at the end of the day. If you eat nothing but crap food, you're going to feel crappy and that's going to affect your mental ability and your ability to deal with stress.

Whenever your diet starts to slip, the stress of the food affects your mental decisions and how you look at things, so you can't be as productive as you should be. The way you want to be all the time is harder because you just can't fight the chemical nature of your body. Making sure that you know how to identify your triggers, like there might be a particular food or something that you're eating that is affecting you. So, make sure your nutrition is tip top and you won't have to worry about stress too much.

Exercise is so great for stress management. A lot of people go to the gym after a big day of work and just sweat out the big work out or whatever they need to feel better. This is a good release, stress release and it is done it in a way that's productive.

Exercise might not be the one for you; it might just be taking a bath or sitting down quietly reading a book. Anything that you need to do to move your body is going to help to leave you out that stress.

The physical stress is of big importance so we can have some good days. We just don't want to have too much bad exercise, too much intensity or too much of a burden that's going to make your stress level go up. So, exercise within your means and do what makes you feel happy and relaxed.

A mental exercise is to revisit your goals and think positively. Don't just think positively for the sake of it. Give yourself reasons to be happy and look for positive things in situations and then make positive choices when it comes down to what you need to do.

To sum up there are good and bad stress. We need to balance all our stress to get results.

Chapter Nine Sleep Rest and Recovery

Sleep patterns, rest, recovery and why it is so important. You might just think it's just a matter of going to bed, but there's a lot more to it than that.

Circadian Rhythm

What we are going to look at is what we call the circadian rhythm. There is a Circadian Rhythm in all animals and creatures on earth, particularly those that are on land and mammals. Not so much things that are in the sea, because they're not affected by the moon and sun except for the tides.

There are two types of animals, either a diurnal, awake and active during the day, or a nocturnal which means that they're awake and active during the night. Now, human beings are diurnal, which means when the sun comes up we wake up; the sun goes down, we go to rest and it goes into loop.

In a perfect world, you'll get up when the sun rises. What happens is whenever we see light or whenever we see sun it triggers off stress, quarters off mainly and that's to wake us up and out of bed and become active.

Evolution and the likes say that if you were asleep during the middle of the day and there's a predator around, we would be lunch. That is why we need to be awake and alert. This is not the case now, but that is ingrained in us as creatures, as animals, so we need to respect that.

We need to understand the signs behind it, so that we can actually give ourselves the adequate rest, repair, and recovery where it's supposed to be. What may happen is that a lot of people will get up at 6am, they'll get through the whole day, and 6pm is just when they're getting home. Usually what they'll do is they'll go into this rest and recovery period usually until 10pm at the latest maybe later.

This is when they're actually starting to think about going to bed or actually getting into bed. This cuts into a huge chunk of our rest and recovery period, because essentially the sun's gone down, so in nature we should start to do the same.

We should start winding down and getting ready for bed. Now, what happens is we've got to cram in getting the kids ready for bed, going out to the gym, going shopping. We're going to cram all these things into this little space of time where we should be resting and winding down.

Working Shifts

For some people this gets even worse. People that work shifts for instance, they're getting up a different time and going to bed at different time. There's a huge chunk of time where the Circadian Rhythm is out of sync. If you're a shift worker, and you feel like you are chronically tired all the time that's because you're robbing yourself of that natural Circadian Rhythm, which we need to be in balance and to have good quality of life.

If you are a shift worker and you can't lose weight or you've got crappy health, or you just feel bad, the only way around this is to not be a shift worker anymore. It's pretty much that simple, because you cannot combat our Circadian Rhythm.

Anything that you do that is in conflict with the Circadian Rhythm and you're going to pay the consequences. If you're a shift worker you go to bed late, get up early. They never actually see balance and rhythm within the scope of the sunrise, sunset and find it really hard to lose weight. Even if they're in the right weight, but just chronically tired all the time, no energy and this is the reason why.

Best Results

What can we do to make the most of it and get the best results? Well, ideally, if you can get up at the same time and go to bed at the same time every day, that's going to be great, a really great start. Try and get to bed by 10:30 at the latest.

When I say get to bed, I mean you need to be asleep by 10:30 every night. That means getting ready to go to bed at 9:30 and then have an hour of winding down in bed and actually drifting off to sleep by 10:30. Now, another thing that we can do is be aware of the things that are beneficial for our sleep and wake pattern.

Good food, low light, no bright lights before bed, plenty of water, and avoid stimulants. If you do these things and make a conscious effort to go to bed and sleep by 10:30, after a couple of days you're going to start to feel a lot better. Your energy level is going to be increased, which will help you do everything else you need to do to get the results you want. Things to watch out for are things like caffeine, sugar, coffee, and tea.

Any of these things before bed or even after lunch can have a stimulating effect and keep your quarters all high, when it should be starting to get lower. All these quarters are the sun, wake up, stress, and activity. Darkness means rest, repair, recovery, and generally that's how the Circadian Rhythm works.

Next Step

Now you are going to jot down a few things that you feel like as when your bedtime is. If you've noticed anything that popped up here like your sleep patterns write them down. Then we will review what actually happens during the sleep cycle and why it's important to get it in between the rhythm.

Let's look at what happens during the 6am to 6pm cycle every day. We've got the bad cycle and the good cycle. If you've got a good cycle, 6am you wake up. You're going to do all your work in the first part of the day, and then towards the end of the evening or towards getting to 6pm, you're starting to decline.

This is the time where all your stressful activity is. Your quarters' all high, you're doing a lot of stuff, working doing your daily routine and you don't expect it to be high. Then, when we get down to 6pm, we've knocked off work and come home.

Your recovery period starts now after 6pm; it's starting to get dark. If you're respecting the Circadian Rhythm and you're going to bed somewhere between 10 and 10:30 pm, allows the appropriate time to be spent in the recovery phase, particularly while you're asleep.

We can split this up into another part. We've got physical repair and then we've got mental repair. You want to have almost an equal balance in terms of where you're spending your time. Between 6am and 10:30pm is the time spent sleeping and 6pm to 10:30pm is spent winding down.

You can see why there is a small amount of stressful activity during the winding down time. Compare this to a disrupted sleep cycle. You wake up and you're in a stressful state for over twelve hours as compared to one which is only six hours or so.

You might be able to get a little bit more depending on what time you get to bed, but for the same time period. Yes, there's a huge difference in rest and recovery.

Like previously we talked about stress with the seesaw. You've got huge amount of time where you're in a high or high stress state, you're having disrupted sleep and then a small rest period. Imagine doing these seven days a week, just over and over and over and over again. I'm sure you've been there before and you've had this sort of feeling.

This is pretty much what's going on. What we need to recognize and need to do is start to shift more into a healthier pattern. If you're not working different shifts, then you've got plenty of time to do this. Really start to lock in that morning wake up time and bedtime every night. Avoid your stimulants and make a conscious effort to get to bed early. Over time, this will start to reset itself and then everything will start to come into balance.

You get the idea of why this can put the brakes on your progress and why you won't lose any weight. You might find it hard or you may just generally not feel very well. The key things to focus on are going to bed by 10:30pm, lots of water, eat well, and manage your stress. All these things will help to manage your stress and help you feel better.

Everything kind of collides together and that's why it's so important to have the combined approach and understanding all these different factors.

Chapter 10 Digestion And Food Intolerance

Welcome to chapter 10, we're going to talk about digestion and intolerance, food intolerance. What is digestion and what intolerance is all about?

Essentially, digestion is something that's often overlooked and forgotten about when it comes to lifestyle change and designing your program. When we think of digestion, everybody eats; everybody has to remove waste from their body.

So the digestive process is the part in the middle where we extract nutrients and basically get all our energy and nutrients from. Everything that we've talked about up until this point has an effect on how well food goes in, and then how it's digested through your body.

So the first step in the process is really the choice that you make in terms of what you're putting into your body in the first place and how's that going to affect your digestive system.

Intolerance

We've already mentioned intolerance in the previous weeks, about the problems that can come with intolerance. Yes, Gluten and dairy, let's call them triggers. So gluten, dairy, and your trigger foods are going to be the ones that are actually going to make you bloated, have poor digestion, and then mal-absorption of your nutrients.

Now, there are extreme cases where you might develop a disorder or a disease like Celiac disease or something like that from gluten in particular and this can be quite dangerous. But, for people that are intolerant, there's a big difference between intolerant and allergic.

Intolerant means that you're not going to die from eating it, but there are certain triggers or certain combinations of food which can actually flare up symptoms like bloating, cramping, and skin breakouts.

All these symptoms that happen in your digestive system is a reflection of what's going on the inside versus what's going on the outside. A good way to describe the intolerance that you might have and how your digestion plays out is to do a little timeline.

Timeline To Intolerance

We've got the timeline of let's say 21 days and you start at day zero. From zero to about 7 days would be considered good. Then between 7 days and 14 days you may have minor symptoms like a pimple, bad breather, or bad smelling gas. When these symptoms get more serious, then you will be in the 14 days to 21 days and have passed the trigger level.

This is when you know your intolerance can turn to something a bit more painful and a bit more severe.

What happens is we breakdown our days to what we are eating. If we're eating gluten, for example, or dairy or something that we're intolerant to and normally don't eat but rarely and we're not getting any symptoms.

Okay, happy days! Yes, we can eat bread and obviously its gluten because it's one of the major ones. What happens is this person is going along, saying okay, I've been eating bread and nothing's been happening.

Let's throw in some alcohol. Let's try some dairy and then there might be a lot of trigger foods, something high in salicylate, amine for example. Amine has to do with the ripening and the composition of some fruits and vegetables when they're high in salicylate, which requires you to have intolerance and responses.

What happens is you peak over after a period of maybe 7 days, it could be 21 days, could be within the same day. But generally, what you're doing is you're layering in intolerance above intolerance, over and over and then eventually you'll get a spike and then a symptom. This might actually happen down at the 21 day level depending on what you're eating.

If you were this person you could not safely say that it was the milk that did it, or the bread that did it, or the alcohol, or the sugar, or the salicylate. Because you have obviously no clue what triggered it.

It's a combination of everything stacking up on top of each other until you get a symptom. I'm eating healthy, but I'm still feeling like crap and my digestion's terrible, and I've got low energy. Your salicylate and amine consumption are pretty neglected and not understood as well and they can affect your digestion, intolerance and how you feel. So, you need to go on an elimination diet where you start cutting out food.

Elimination Diet

Let's say you decide to cut out gluten for a whole week. More information on the elimination diet that you can get from the API hospital, I'll leave a link. There's a little book you can buy and download that goes into it a lot more and definitely explains how you can actually conduct the elimination diet.

The diet is done in various stages where you cut out a ton of food and have very basic food groups to eat from and then slowly reintroduce new foods. If you got kids with allergies this is the best way to eliminate certain foods. We're trying to establish a baseline diet where you get no symptoms. Then you slowly reintroduce bread and if you get a symptom then you take it out again. Introduce dairy, maybe you got a symptom and then now you know that it's one or the other.

Whatever that food might be, you may need some assistance with a nutritionist. We've got some nutritionists on our blog that we recommend and work with around Australia for your convenience.

Generally, if you eat something and then half an hour to twenty hours later you start to feel ordinary, you can sort of intuitively know that food is okay, or maybe this isn't the best food for me because it's making me feel like crap.

Think back to your food diary, you would notice that pattern because you eat something, get a symptom, look back and then just see what food is was. You can now see how this all ties together.

Review

Keep track and get an idea of what your body is actually doing and how it's affecting you, then what you can do to change it. You might need to reach out to get a professional to help you, particularly someone who deals in salicylate and amines, and elimination diets. Depending on how intolerant or allergic you might be, you may need to see someone.

However, if you're just a little bit intolerant like most people, generally, you can recognize your trigger foods and then take steps to minimize your exposure to it. This is going to help your digestion tremendously, because what we need to do is think about detoxing as well. That's what digestion is all about, detoxing and getting your nutrients.

Everything we've talked about now, especially, sleep and stress affect all of these. If you don't have a good night sleep you can't actually actively digest, detox, and get your nutrition. What happens is they get cut and don't function properly and this slows down your metabolism. Then, you can become lethargic and tired. You don't have much nutrition on board, so therefore you can't function properly.

Tips for your digestion are to make sure you're absorbing your food correctly and you're monitoring your intolerance. Use your food diary and look back and see if you've got a trigger and identify if that's something that you can remove. You want to have plenty of water. You want to always eat slowly and in a relaxed way.

You've got to avoid stimulants like tea, coffee, sugar, soft drink, and all that crap food. Alcohol is another one and medical drugs. If you have to take medication, it is going to affect your digestion. Digestion can become stressful, as we talked about stress in the previous week and how it all summates into one big stress picture. If your digestion is under stress your body doesn't actually have the time to sit down, break down, and digest all your food correctly. Problems with your digestion affect your energy levels. Everything affects each other.

At this stage, you're probably distinctly going to start to notice some of these things. What we talked about beforehand in terms of how digestion works is what you really need to know to take it to that next level and just use your food diary and your common sense. Start to notice if you eat something that made you feel a bit ordinary, make a note of it.

Remove it from your diet for a couple of days or even a week. If you start to feel better then obviously, reintroduce it. If the symptoms flare up again you can safely say that that's a problem food. This does take a little bit of trial and error, because you've got to try food, take them out, and reintroduce them slowly.

If you're following the clean eating plan, it's going to give you a good basis to start with and then it's not so difficult. You will get to a point where you design your own meal plan, just by feel, and then that's probably the best way. Look at it as a life time process, because now you've got education behind. You know what's happening rather than just that you're powerless to fix it.

So, pay attention to your digestion and use your food diary. Notice if you're getting triggers on certain foods and then look at eliminating them for five to seven days. I'll leave some more resources and some links that you can look at that will help you with the elimination diet in particular. Where you can get a copy of that and how you can find someone if you need a little bit extra help.

Chapter Eleven Bringing It All Together

After being on any type of weight loss program we want to keep the results we have achieved. The good habits and new beliefs you will have learned do not need to end once you stop dieting or exercising.

So making sure you keep that 9 step process in mind will help you stay on track as you enter what we would call the maintenance phase. All the hard work is completed its now just up to you to carry on doing the right things If you eat well, do well you'll be well. If you eat great, be great, do great you get the idea.

You are what you eat. When it comes to your food and diet planning is key. Taking things slow and also doing one thing at a time working your way through the 9 step system. I built it out this way to help you see the path to results and where you may need to start changing you habits.

We have covered a lot so far and it can be hard to try and do everything at once. The basics we have covered should help you get 80% the way to your results. The other 20% will require you to take action follow the process. And of course make small changes as you go.

Doing the basic's every day like getting to bed on time, eating those three to five meals, eating clean, exercising three to five times a week, staying focused, staying consistent, staying positive.

That's pretty much all you need to do to have lasting success. It's all the stuff we've talked about beforehand all ads up to getting you the knowledge to achieve the lasting change.

Also re visit and revise your goals regularly, make sure they are still relevant to you and they matter. It's ok to change your goals in line with how you want to live. It's important to remember it's about you not anybody else.

Regularly, and track your progress. You will be truly on your way to keeping these results and building that good solid habit.

It's never a straight line to get to your goals; it's always all over the place. Now there are going to be times where you feel this way. And its ok just remembers the earlier chapters and work your way through the system to see where you're stuck.

When you try and change something or learn something new it's a process it's always going to be ups and downs and things that you have to deal with that pop up.

Take your time and the results will come.

Let this just be the beginning for you and remember we are here to help. If you have any questions or need any help please reach out and contact me on the website.

We have other products and programs that will help you get the results faster like my online meal planner program or even some one on one coaching. There are plenty of way's we can help you.

Thanks again for reading this eBook. I hope you got a lot out of it and it will help get the weight loss results you deserve.

www.ingramcontent.com/pod-product-compliance
Lightning Source LLC
Chambersburg PA
CBHW070600290526
45790CB00002B/737